_____

I have put it off long enough. I am ready to stop giving a fuck and start living my best life.

If found, please . . .

return ⭕

shred ⭕

burn ⭕

do yourself a favor
and buy your own
f**king copy ⭕

Also by Sarah Knight

The Life-Changing Magic of Not Giving a F**k

Get Your Sh*t Together

Get Your Sh*t Together Journal

You Do You

Calm the F**k Down

Calm the F**k Down Journal

F**k No!

The Life-Changing Magic of Not Giving a F**k Journal

Practical ways to care less
and get more

SARAH KNIGHT

Quercus

Not giving a fuck: the basics

- **Not giving a fuck means taking care of yourself first**—like affixing your own oxygen mask before helping others.

- **Not giving a fuck means allowing yourself to say no.** I don't want to. I don't have time. I can't afford it.

- **Not giving a fuck—crucially—means releasing yourself from the worry, anxiety, fear, and guilt associated with saying no,** allowing you to stop spending time you don't have with people you don't like doing things you don't want to do.

- **Not giving a fuck means reducing mental clutter** and eliminating annoying people and things from your life, freeing up space to truly enjoy all of the things you *do* give a fuck about.

This might sound selfish, and it is. But it also creates a better world for everyone around you.

You'll stop worrying about all the things you *have* to do and start focusing on the things you *want* to do. You'll be happier and more carefree at work; your colleagues and clients will benefit. You'll be better rested and more fun around friends. You might spend more time with your family—or you might spend less, making those moments you do share all the more precious. And you'll have more time, energy, and/or money to devote to living your best life.

The people who embrace the life-changing magic of not giving a fuck are WINNING.

You want to be one of these people, don't you?

I thought so. Let's get started.

What it is

In case it is not patently obvious, this journal is based on a book I wrote called *The Life-Changing Magic of Not Giving a Fuck: How to Stop Spending Time You Don't Have Doing Things You Don't Want to do with People You Don't Like*. You may have noticed the similarities between the title of my book/journal and the title of a book by Japanese author Marie Kondo: *The Life-Changing Magic of Tidying Up*. Good eye! That was intentional.

In 2015, after quitting my corporate job and feeling rather liberated by all the fucks I no longer gave to conference calls, useless paperwork, and commuting on the underground B.O. factory that is the New York City subway, I set out to write an affectionate parody of an internationally bestselling tidying guide. Ms. Kondo's book was about cleaning out your house; mine would be about cleaning out your *mind*. It would poke gentle fun at her methods—such as when she instructs readers to ask if a particular object "sparks joy" before deciding whether to get rid of it—while illustrating how one can similarly rid one's brain (and subsequently one's calendar and credit card bill) of unnecessary crap by learning how to just not give a fuck about stuff that *annoys* you.

See what I did there?

In *The Life-Changing Magic of Not Giving a Fuck Journal*, you'll be getting all of the best tips, tricks, and techniques from the original book, plus new exercises, and less of my scintillating personal story but more room to sort through your own bullshit.

I hope you brought pencils.

Oh, and a giant black marker. We'll get to that later, but do go out and buy one if you don't already have seventeen of them lurking in the junk drawer like I do.

In the first part of the journal, I'll explain some fundamental concepts on your journey to giving fewer, better fucks—including mental decluttering; joy vs. annoy; the Language of Opinion; and my two-step NotSorry Method. Then we'll move into the practical side of things. I'll teach you how to make a Fuck Budget, and you'll work on moving stuff in and out of it as you see fit.

Oh, and do you like making lists? THEN YOU ARE IN LUCK. Lists galore, I tell you!

Seriously, pencils. Plural.

Who it's for

If you're like me, you've been giving too many fucks about too many things for too long. You're overextended, overburdened, stressed out, and anxious. Maybe even legit panic-stricken about your commitments. That's no way to live. And if you continue on your current path—then at the end of each day, or week, or month, you're bound to find yourself scraping the bottom of your own personal fuck barrel.

Which is when you'll realize that all those fucks you gave away were for the benefit of everyone but YOU.

It's time to flip the script, reverse the curse, and stop giving all of your fucks to all the wrong things for all the wrong reasons.

Rather than blindly pressing forward and saying *Yes, YES, YES!!!* to all of the people and things that demand your time, energy, and/or money, the first thing you should be asking yourself before uttering that dirty little three-letter word is, *Do I really give a fuck?*

This journal will help you get to your answer—and then help you put it into practice.

A word on the F-word

In the parlance of my No Fucks Given Guides series, "giving a fuck" has two linked meanings.

- To "give a fuck" means to care about something. You like watching *Jeopardy!* at 7:00p.m. every night? Then you give a fuck about *Jeopardy!*

- But "giving a fuck" also means literally *giving* your fucks to that thing. Your time, energy, and money—henceforth known as your "fuck bucks"—should ideally be dispensed in service to things you care (i.e., give a fuck) about. You spend your time watching *Jeopardy!*, your energy making sure you're home in time for the show, and perhaps your money on the cable bill that funnels Alex Trebek's endearing smarm into your home.

Conversely, when you DO NOT care about something and DO NOT give your fucks to that thing, you *gain* time, energy, and/or money to spend on other stuff. Hence the subtitle of this very journal: "practical ways to care less and get more."

Later, we'll press the fuck bucks analogy to its logical conclusion by making a Fuck Budget. But first, allow me to introduce you to the method that underpins my entire *oeuvre* . . .

Mental decluttering and
the NotSorry Method

Just as Marie Kondo has her "KonMari Method" for decluttering and reorganizing your physical space, I have my "NotSorry Method" for decluttering and reorganizing *your mental space* by giving fewer, better fucks. Remember that (among other things) not giving a fuck means not giving your time, energy, and/or money to things that annoy you—so you'll have more resources left to spend on things that bring you joy.

The NotSorry Method has two steps:

1. Decide what you don't give a fuck about
2. Don't give a fuck about those things

And if you complete these steps using a combination of honesty and politeness, then you will have done nothing wrong, have nothing to feel guilty about, and have nothing to apologize for.

You will be quite literally "not sorry."

THE
NOTSORRY METHOD

STEP 1:

DECIDE WHAT YOU DON'T GIVE A FUCK ABOUT.

STEP 2:

DON'T GIVE A FUCK ABOUT THOSE THINGS.

* * *

But before
you can take
Step 1…

...you need to
stop giving a fuck
about what other
people think.

Feelings vs. opinions

If the NotSorry Method unlocks the door to life-changing magic, not giving a fuck about what other people think is how you get on the property in the first place. It paves the way toward taking Step 1 (deciding not to give a fuck); and then you can express your decisions in a positive and productive way when taking Step 2 (not giving a fuck).

Plus, you can do it without offending or enraging anyone! (Unless you really want to offend or enrage; sometimes that can be fun.)

But first things first. You know that shame and guilt you feel when you're trying so hard to not give a fuck? Please listen when I say: it's usually not because you are *wrong* to not give that fuck. It's because you're worried about *what other people might think* about your decision.

And guess what? You have no control over what other people think. For God's sake, you have a hard enough time figuring out what YOU think!

Believing that you have any control over what other people think—and wasting your fucks on that pursuit—is futile. It is a recipe for failure on a grand fucking scale.

Nope. When it comes to how your fuck-giving affects other people, all you can control is your behavior with regard to their feelings, not their opinions.

But I can't possibly stop worrying about what other people think. It's programmed into my DNA!

Ah, but your DNA can only take you so far. In order to live your best life, you're going to have to hack the system.

There are two reasons you tend to give a fuck about what other people think:

1. Because you don't want to *be* a bad person
2. Because you don't want to *look like* a bad person

You should, of course, continue to give a fuck about what other people think as it pertains to their feelings (i.e., Are you going to actively hurt those feelings by not giving a fuck about the situation at hand?).

But be honest—you know full well when you're hurting someone's feelings. Don't be an asshole.

10 THINGS ASSHOLES
DON'T GIVE A FUCK ABOUT

Other people's personal space

Making you wait

Talking in the train's quiet car

Littering

Tipping appropriately

Causing gross smells in confined areas

Using turn signals properly

Blocking the escalator

Cleaning up after their pets

Being perceived as assholes

What I'm saying is, you do not have to give a fuck about what others think when it comes to their opinions—opinions which YOU CANNOT CONTROL, remember? And if you can learn to speak to people in the Language of Opinion (opinions being things we are all entitled to have), I think you will find it both disarming and relatively easy.

You can sidestep the prospect of hurt feelings entirely when you view your conflict through the lens of simple, emotionless opinion.

You will neither *be* an asshole nor *look like* an asshole.

And then you can stop worrying about what other people think.

In a few pages, we'll practice speaking in the Language of Opinion; but first let's discuss the twin pillars of the NotSorry Method:

HONESTY

and

POLITENESS

Honesty and politeness: a dynamic duo

I can't overemphasize that, when done correctly, not giving a fuck does *not* mean "being an asshole."

In order to achieve peak NotSorry, you need to conduct yourself honorably. After all, you don't want to lose friends; you simply want to get more enjoyment (and less annoyance) out of the time you spend with your friends. You don't want to alienate family; you want to coexist peacefully with them at times that are mutually convenient for all involved. Etcetera.

And through years of rigorous fieldwork, I've found that a combination of honesty and politeness results in the smoothest transition to fewer fucks given AND fewer relationships destroyed.

See, honesty alone isn't going to cut it, and neither is politeness all by itself. You could be extremely honest but very rude, which means someone deserves an apology. Or you could be superpolite and a total fucking liar—and a tidbit of fibbing is one thing, but if you get caught in a monster lie, I guarantee you're going to be sorry, which kinda defeats the purpose of the entire method.

The key is to blend honesty and politeness into a perfect combination, like Siegfried and Roy, Hall and Oates, and Batman and Robin.

Together they're capable of making magic, hitting all the right notes, and saving the day. And they never fail to complement each other, even if one shines a little brighter at times, or gets mauled by a tiger.

TRANSLATION SKILLS: AN EXERCISE

On this page, I've provided a list of potentially feelings-hurting, apology-requiring statements. They may be honest, but they fall well short of polite.

LANGUAGE OF FEELINGS

1. I'm not coming to your dinner party on Tuesday because I hate your boyfriend.

2. I won't participate in the group Spice Girls costume because I think we will look like a bunch of sad old tramps.

3. No, I don't want to donate to your stupid pet cause.

4. I don't have time to listen to you prattle on about meaningless shit.

5. I've got better things to do than go on a double-decker bus tour of downtown St. Louis with my in-laws.

6. I don't have enough money to waste it going out for drinks with coworkers I don't even like.

TRANSLATION SKILLS: AN EXERCISE

On this page, you get to practice translating my statements into the Language of Opinion. Like so:

LANGUAGE OF OPINION

1. Example: Tuesdays are tough nights for me to go out.

2. Example: I don't think the Spice Girls are really my style.

3. ....

   ....

4. ....

   ....

5. ....

   ....

6. ....

   ....

TRANSLATION SKILLS: AN EXERCISE
(part two)

Now let's move on to things YOU don't give a fuck about. Use this page to write honestly about them, without concern for other people's feelings.

LANGUAGE OF FEELINGS

1. ....

....

2. ....

....

3. ....

....

4. ....

....

5. ....

....

6. ....

....

TRANSLATION SKILLS: AN EXERCISE
(part two cont.)

———————————

And use this page to translate those statements into the simple, emotionless Language of Opinion.

LANGUAGE OF OPINION

1.

2.

3.

4.

5.

6.

Visualize it!

Before we move on, I want you to take a minute and do a free-form visualization of all the stuff that you currently feel pressured—by friends, family, society, or even your own twisted sense of obligation—to give a fuck about.

These could include, but are not limited to; matching your belt to your handbag, LinkedIn, eating local, hot yoga, paleo diets, the Harry Potter books, Kombucha, "trending," podcasts, ponchos-as-fashion, the Ballet, Bret Easton Ellis, fair-trade coffee, the Cloud, other people's children, sanctimonious Christians, understanding China's economy, #catsofinstagram, *The Voice*, your father's new wife, and/or Burning Man.

Felling a tad ill, are you? Jittery, nauseous, anxious? Pissed off?

Good, then it's working.

Now visualize how happy and carefree you would be if you stopped giving all those fucks.

Hot yoga? Don't give a downward fuck! The Cloud? Fucks not found. And #catsofinstagram? Sorry, you're all outta fucks, meow.

Doesn't that feel so much better? I'm telling you, if you follow my NotSorry Method for not giving a fuck, your spirit will be lighter, your calendar will be clearer, and your time and energy will be spent on only the things and people you enjoy.

It's life-changing. Swear to God.

STEP 1:

DECIDE WHAT YOU DON'T GIVE A FUCK ABOUT.

JOY

vs.

ANNOY

Joy vs. Annoy

In order to complete Step 1 of the NotSorry Method—deciding what you don't give a fuck about—I recommend asking yourself not what brings you joy, but what ANNOYS you. This is because I find that extricating myself from a *current* state of annoyance is more motivating than reaching a *potential* state of joy.

(Also, "joy" and "annoy" are opposing concepts that rhyme, and as I mentioned, this entire gig started out as a parody. Get used to it, because there's more silly-yet-practical wordplay where that came from.)

For now, use the next couple of pages to keep a running list of stuff that annoys you. Entries could take the form of activities, events, concepts, or even people. Don't hold back! We'll revisit this list later when it comes time to practice budgeting your fucks.

STUFF THAT ANNOYS ME

MORE STUFF THAT ANNOYS ME

EVEN MORE STUFF THAT ANNOYS ME

P.S.: Now might be a good time to think about where you're going to hide this journal while you're not using it.

One person's joy can be
another person's annoy.
And that's okay.

Your fucks are *yours*—to
value and prioritize and give
as you see fit.

The Holy Fucking Trinity

TIME

ENERGY

MONEY

The number of fucks
you personally have to give
is a finite and precious
commodity.

What's in your Fuck Budget?

You know how satisfying it is when you spend a few months saving up for something you really want to buy, and then you go to the store and you have the money in hand and you walk out with a new snowboard or whatever?

In that moment, you're probably not thinking about all the things you sacrificed over the past hundred days in order to accumulate the funds necessary to pay for that snowboard. But you did sacrifice. Maybe you went without your Dunkin' Donuts Angus Steak and Egg Sandwich every day for three months. Or maybe you took on more hours working *at* Dunkin' Donuts to make extra cash (thereby sacrificing free time).

Either way, you had a goal—to save the cost of the snowboard—and you stuck to a budget relative to how much money you had to save and/or how many hours you had to work to achieve your goal.

I suggest you implement a similar budget for your fucks.

BALANCING YOUR FUCK BUDGET:
AN EXERCISE

When you think about it, life is a series of yes-or-no choices, fucks given and fucks withheld.

Choose five of the things that annoy you from the list you made on pages 28–30. Put those in the left-hand column. This is stuff you DON'T want to spend your time, energy, and money on.

In the right-hand column, write down something you DO want to spend your fuck bucks on—specifically, something you could do if you freed up time, energy, and money from the left-hand column. Like so:

Stuff I don't want to spend time on (annoy)	Stuff I do want to spend time on (joy)
Working out	Sleeping

Stuff I don't want to spend energy on (annoy)	Stuff I do want to spend energy on (joy)
Worrying about the threat of a nuclear Iran	Fighting climate change

Stuff I don't want to spend money on (annoy)	Stuff I do want to spend money on (joy)
"Glamping"	Laser hair removal

TIME

Sometimes all you want is a free hour to take a leisurely bath and clip your toenails. By not giving a fuck about making an appearance at your neighbor's vegan BBQ, you get back that hour. Soak it in!

Stuff I don't want to spend time on (annoy)	Stuff I do want to spend time on (joy)

ENERGY

Sometimes you wish you could get up and go to the gym at six in the morning when no one else is watching. By not giving a fuck about attending someone's ill-conceived ten o'clock Tuesday-night dinner party (WTF?), you can stay sober, rest up, and be bright-eyed and bushy-tailed on Wednesday for your date with the elliptical machine.

Stuff I don't want to spend time on (annoy)	Stuff I do want to spend time on (joy)

MONEY

Sometimes you want that Caribbean vacation so bad you get sand in your shorts just thinking about it. By not giving a fuck about your grade-school friend's wedding that you don't understand why you were invited to in the first place, you can march on over to JetBlue.com and reallocate the thousand dollars you totally would have spent on it before reading this journal, and you can do it with a clear conscience. NotSorry all the way to the Virgin Islands, baby.

Stuff I don't want to spend money on (annoy)	Stuff I do want to spend money on (joy)

Don't say yes right away.

Instead, take a moment to question not only whether you give a fuck (i.e., care) *about* something but also whether it deserves a fuck i.e. your time, energy, and/or money given to it as a line item on your Fuck Budget.

Stop. Calculate. And maybe don't give that fuck.

A fucking recap

The life-changing magic of not giving a fuck is all about prioritizing. Joy over annoy. Choice over obligation. Opinions vs. feelings. Sticking to a budget. Eyes on the prize.

Let's review the basics—the tools and processes for Deciding Whether or Not to Give a Fuck so you can proceed to Give or Not Give a Fuck:

- Does the fuck you're about to give (or not give) affect only you? Or others?

- If the former, you are *way* ahead of the game!

- If the latter, you must first stop giving a fuck about what other people think, before you can move on to not giving a fuck about the matter at hand.

- In order to do that, consider their *opinions* separately from their *feelings*.

- Don't be an asshole.

- Now consult your Fuck Budget: What is that fuck worth to you? Do you really want to give it?

- If the answer is yes, then by all means, go for it! But if the answer is no, proceed in an honest and polite fashion toward not giving a fuck and being 100 percent, bona fide NotSorry.

In case you're one of those visual learners, here is a flowchart for determining whether you give a fuck. Feel free to refer back to it as you journal on.

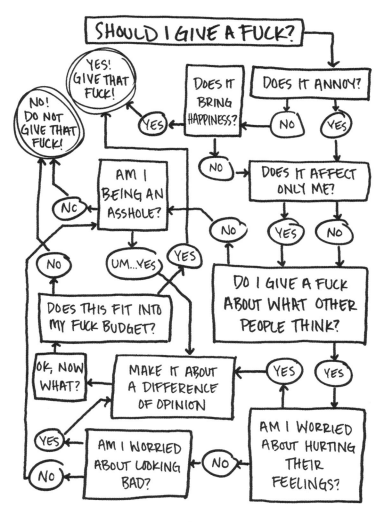

Personal policies

A "personal policy" is a concept that will serve you well in your pursuit of no-fucks-given, best-life-livin'. Here's how it works:

If there's something I don't give a fuck about, but that exists in a gray area of potentially hurting someone else's feelings no matter how honest and polite I am about expressing it, I simply chalk my position up to a "personal policy."

As in: "I have a personal policy against donating to Kickstarter campaigns, because if I donate to one, I feel like I have to donate to them all. I just can't afford it, and if I had to choose, I wouldn't want anyone I love to think I value them more or less than anyone else."

Imagine you're on the other end of that response. You might get a little huffy for a hot second, but can you really . . . argue? No, you cannot. At least, not without being an asshole.

Zing!

Now you try:

"I have a personal policy against ...., because if I .... one, I feel like I have to .... them all. I just don't have the [time/energy/money] and if I had to choose, I wouldn't want anyone I love to think I value them more or less than anyone else."

"I have a personal policy against ...., because if I .... one, I feel like I have to .... them all. I just don't have the [time/energy/money] and if I had to choose, I wouldn't want anyone I love to think I value them more or less than anyone else."

"I have a personal policy against ...., because if I .... one, I feel like I have to .... them all. I just don't have the [time/energy/money] and if I had to choose, I wouldn't want anyone I love to think I value them more or less than anyone else."

There, that wasn't so hard, was it? Ideally, a personal policy functions like an onside kick in American football: surprising, impossible to defend, and if done right, a total game-changer.

OTHER THINGS YOU*
MIGHT HAVE A PERSONAL
POLICY AGAINST

Breakfast meetings

Karaoke

Potluck dinners

Changing diapers

Driving more than four hours
round trip in the same day

Bob Dylan

Raw fish

Snow

---

* Actually, these are mine.
You can write yours
on the next page.

THINGS I MIGHT DEVELOP
A PERSONAL POLICY AGAINST

....

....

....

....

....

....

....

....

....

Your mind is a barn

Let's take it back to mental decluttering, the process by which you'll sort your fucks into those that bring joy and those that annoy.

Just like physical decluttering, this is a process of discarding stuff you don't want or need, and then organizing what you have left into some semblance of a happier, more tranquil existence. In both cases, you've got to know what you're dealing with. You have to take inventory.

We're going to do this by visualizing your mind as a gigantic barn full of crap. It contains all the stuff you're being asked to give a fuck about right now, whether you want to or have to, or not. (This joint is a big fucking mess. Have you seen *Hoarders*? I think I'm getting a rash.)

The problem is, most of us only poke our heads into the barn every once in a while, and never get past the mountain of shit piled up just inside the door—much less do anything about the rest of it. NOT GOOD ENOUGH.

You're going to have to get all the way inside and really fucking own up to it before you have any hope of clearing it out, a process which may lead to a condition I call "Fuck Overload."

Fuck Overload

When you confront all of the stuff you're
expected to give a fuck about all at once, your gut
may clench, your bowels may roil, and your head
and heart may begin to pound. But do not despair,
for THIS IS THE WHOLE POINT. We are aiming
for Fuck Overload here, people. I believe you need
to experience it in order to fully recognize the time,
energy, and/or money you're spending on
your fucks—and to get excited about
pruning them once and for all.

Soon, you'll begin taking inventory of your mental barn.
You will identify every fuck being demanded of you; you
will acknowledge it and size it up and think good and
hard about whether you really want and need to give it.

Do this once and thoroughly, and you'll have a method to
free yourself for life, even as the fucks demanded of you
change over time. You won't let that mental clutter pile
up again, because you'll have the tools and perspective to
keep the things you don't give a fuck about from winding
up in there in the first place. BOOM.

Okay, fine. We don't want to go *overboard* on Fuck Overload. In order to make taking mental barn inventory a smidge easier, I've devised four categories of potential fuck-giving:

THINGS

WORK

FRIENDS, ACQUAINTANCES,
AND STRANGERS

FAMILY

Together, these categories constitute the vast miasma of people and things that you could potentially stop giving a fuck about, but we're going to work through them one at a time.

THINGS come first in your pursuit of not giving a fuck because they are inanimate and can't talk back.

Then WORK, because it provokes some feeling of bitterness and resentment in nearly every person I know, which is a good motivator.

Then FRIENDS, ACQUAINTANCES, AND STRANGERS once you've got your sea legs.

FAMILY comes last in your study of not giving a fuck, for what should be obvious reasons. That shit is hard. (But not impossible—I promise!)

Let's begin . . .

THINGS

This category deals with inanimate objects and concepts, neither of which possess the irksome feelings and opinions of your fellow human beings, making them the easiest to stop giving a fuck about.

Examples include but are not limited to:

Gardening	Pedicures	Being on time
Gluten	TikTok	"Having it all"
Ice skating	The news	Drinking eight glasses of water per day

(I give a fuck about exactly four of these things, but you do you!)

The next few pages provide space for you to write down all of the things that may be demanding your time, energy, and/or money—regardless of whether or not you want to include them in your Fuck Budget.

Take stock of your mental barn. What are the things that make you sigh involuntarily with pleasure? How about the ones that create a feeling in your stomach evocative of a fork getting stuck in the garbage disposal?

Does it bring joy or does it annoy?

For now, IT DOESN'T MATTER. List 'em all!

THINGS I MAY OR MAY NOT
GIVE A FUCK ABOUT

(an inventory)

THINGS I MAY OR MAY NOT
GIVE A FUCK ABOUT

(an inventory)

....
....
....
....
....
....
....
....
....
....
....
....
....
....
....
....
....
....

THINGS I MAY OR MAY NOT
GIVE A FUCK ABOUT

(an inventory)

THINGS I MAY OR MAY NOT
GIVE A FUCK ABOUT

(an inventory)

THINGS I MAY OR MAY NOT
GIVE A FUCK ABOUT

(an inventory)

_____   _____

_____   _____

_____   _____

_____   _____

_____   _____

_____   _____

_____   _____

_____   _____

_____   _____

_____   _____

_____   _____

_____   _____

_____   _____

Onward, to WORK!

Work

More complicated than the previous category—which simply involves withholding your fucks from inanimate objects/concepts/activities—work is still not quite as fraught as dealing with friends and family, thus making it the logical second point of entry to getting this life-changing magic under way.

Additionally, if you ask a bunch of random people what they hate most in life, lots of them are going to say their jobs, bosses, coworkers, IT departments, or something in that realm. Kind of a wide target.

Luckily, there are plenty of perfectly acceptable ways to reduce the number of fucks you give at work—whether it's bailing on an unnecessary meeting or declining an invitation to a coworker's party—and still continue to remain employed, respected, and even well liked (if you give a fuck about that; see p. 62, "The Likability Vortex").

Imagine there's a set of dented metal file cabinets lining the walls of your barn. Yank out every drawer, one by one, and make a list of all the work-related fucks you find inside. And don't forget your subcategories, such as Bosses, Coworkers, Office Politics, Meetings, Memos, etc.; and then sub-subcategories, such as Coworkers' Feelings, Birthdays, and Sick Pets. You know what I'm going to say . . .

List 'em all!

WORK-RELATED STUFF I MAY OR MAY NOT GIVE A FUCK ABOUT

(an inventory)

WORK-RELATED STUFF I MAY OR MAY NOT GIVE A FUCK ABOUT

(an inventory)

WORK-RELATED STUFF I MAY OR MAY NOT GIVE A FUCK ABOUT

(an inventory)

WORK-RELATED STUFF I MAY OR MAY NOT GIVE A FUCK ABOUT

(an inventory)

WORK-RELATED STUFF I MAY OR MAY NOT GIVE A FUCK ABOUT

(an inventory)

The Likability Vortex

Being liked and being respected are not necessarily the same thing. For one, it's a lot easier to keep your job if you are respected rather than merely liked. I've "liked" plenty of incompetent wastoids in my time, but I wouldn't hire them.

The Likability Vortex occurs when you care more about being liked than about being worthy of respect. You wind up floundering inside a devastating fucknado of your own design.

Why?

Because you can't control whether or not people like you.

You might be a funny person, but your particular sense of humor doesn't jive with someone else's and they won't like you. You might be super-friendly, but others might perceive that as weird and not like you. You might be completely inoffensive, but you remind Helen of her ex-boyfriend AND SHE JUST DOESN'T LIKE YOU.

What you CAN control—by giving your fucks to the aspects of your job that make you damn good at it—is whether you are worthy of others' respect. They may or may not give it to you (they've got their own fucks to budget, after all), but if you're doing a good job, at least *you* know you're worthy.

And if doing a good job means spending more fucks on getting shit done and fewer on whether people like you *while* you're getting it done, then you've escaped the Likability Vortex and the fucknado that comes with it.

Nice work. Take the rest of the day off.

Are you worried that your friends will be mad at you if you just tell them the polite truth?

Then you worry too much.

Friends, acquaintances, and strangers

We love our friends. That's why they *are* our friends. But all relationships are complicated, and sometimes friends get on friends' nerves. I do it all the time, such as when I get drunk and put things on my head and force my friends to take pictures. I realize this gets annoying, but hey, maybe they should leave quietly before I get to my fifth glass of wine! This is precisely why it's important to develop your internal strategy for not giving a fuck when it comes to conflicts that could put significant strain on—or even destroy—a friendship.

The thing is, other people deposit a lot of their fucks in your mental barn. Some of these are short-term storage. Some have been gathering dust in a back corner for years. It doesn't matter—the real question is, how did those fucks get there in the first place?

Oh, that's right. You let them in.

Now you've got to write 'em out.

Use the next few pages to list all of the fucks being demanded of you by your friends, acquaintances, and random strangers. Again, it doesn't matter right now if you do or do not want to give those fucks—just get them all onto the page for now, and we'll sort them out a bit later in the journal.

FRIENDS, ACQUAINTANCES, STRANGERS, AND RELATED ITEMS I MAY OR MAY NOT GIVE A FUCK ABOUT

(an inventory)

FRIENDS, ACQUAINTANCES, STRANGERS, AND RELATED ITEMS I MAY OR MAY NOT GIVE A FUCK ABOUT

(an inventory)

FRIENDS, ACQUAINTANCES, STRANGERS, AND RELATED ITEMS I MAY OR MAY NOT GIVE A FUCK ABOUT

(an inventory)

FRIENDS, ACQUAINTANCES, STRANGERS, AND RELATED ITEMS I MAY OR MAY NOT GIVE A FUCK ABOUT

(an inventory)

FRIENDS, ACQUAINTANCES, STRANGERS, AND RELATED ITEMS I MAY OR MAY NOT GIVE A FUCK ABOUT

(an inventory)

Setting boundaries

In your quest to not be annoyed by friends, acquaintances, and even strangers, you need to set some boundaries around your barn.

Maybe these are invisible boundaries, like those electric shock fences people set up to keep their pets from escaping. Like, let's say that every time you go to a certain couple's house, their giant, slobbery dog tries to lick your crotch like it's full of Alpo, and you want to avoid going there so you can avoid being *annoyed* at your friends by way of their crotch-licking dog. You don't give a fuck about dealing with their dog, but you don't want to tell them this because you suspect it will hurt their feelings. You're so polite!

So you set a private boundary: you invite them to come to you, or suggest neutral hangout spots where your crotch can remain out of harm's way. And if they have a gathering at their house, maybe you get a little tummy ache that night. There's no harm in pleading gastric distress every once in a while to keep a friendship intact.

Sometimes your boundaries can be more obvious, like a tasteful NO TRESPASSING sign, or that fancy coiled wire they string up around prison yards.

For example, early in my development of the NotSorry Method, I was confronted with The Pub Trivia Problem.

NOTSORRY
PRESENTS:

....

The
Pub Trivia
Problem

I have a group of friends who just *loooooove* pub trivia. In Williamsburg! (For those who don't know—Williamsburg, Brooklyn, is a godawful hipster wasteland populated exclusively by mustaches and empty cans of Pabst Blue Ribbon.) When I used to live in New York, they kept asking me to join them and I kept making lame excuses not to go. Then I would have to remember what my excuse was lest I get caught out on Facebook during pub trivia "GETTING MY NAP ON."

But once I embraced NotSorry, instead of racking my brain to come up with yet another lame excuse—and then having to self-police my social media to make sure I didn't get caught in a lie—the next time they asked, I just said, "You know what? I really don't like pub trivia, and I'm not big on Williamsburg either, so my answer to this is always going to be no. I should probably just tell you that now and save us all the Kabuki theater of invitation and regrets."

I erected my fence and it worked like a charm!

Once my friends knew the truth, I felt Liberated with a capital *L*. I was honest and polite, and nobody's feelings got hurt so I didn't have to apologize. I was definitively not sorry.

Plus—major win—I didn't have to go to pub trivia in Williamsburg.

BOUNDARIES: AN EXERCISE

Use the next few pages to write about some times when you failed to set a boundary.

What happened as a result? Did you wind up doing something you didn't want to do? Spending money you couldn't afford? Wasting time you didn't have?

How did it make you feel?

What can you do to keep it from happening again?

BOUNDARIES: AN EXERCISE

BOUNDARIES: AN EXERCISE

BOUNDARIES: AN EXERCISE

BOUNDARIES: AN EXERCISE

IT'S TIME TO
TALK ABOUT THE
MOTHER OF ALL
FUCK-GIVING ...

Family

Oh, family. Oh, *them*.

Like the Tax Office, your family exists to fuck with you. All of those group photos, weddings, bar and bat mitzvahs, christenings, quinceañeras, all-inclusive vacations, group-therapy sessions, right-wing uncles, sibling rivalries, drama, and grudges promote constant, daily fuck-giving.

And like the certain (some might say, inordinately large) percentage of your income that the government reserves for taxes, a certain percentage of your fucks seem to be automatically reserved by your family—many of whom seem to think you *have to* hand them over just because you share DNA. On that, I call bullshit.

After all, one of the central tenets of living your best life is choice over obligation. And as we all know, you don't get to choose your family—so at the very least, you should get to choose *how and why you interact with them.* Right? Right.

This is the last time you'll have to venture inside your mental barn. The family fucks you've been storing in there are likely buried three-deep under a blanket of cobwebs and resentment—but once you dust 'em off and haul those fuckers out into the light, the hard work is done.

So make that final list, and make it count!

FAMILY STUFF I MAY OR MAY NOT GIVE A FUCK ABOUT

(an inventory)

FAMILY STUFF I MAY OR MAY NOT
GIVE A FUCK ABOUT

(an inventory)

A note on in-laws

In-laws are basically a package deal; what you really wanted to ride home off the lot was your spouse, but the dealership threw in some extra people for free. Some of them could wind up being nice perks, like those armrests in the backseat with built-in cup holders; others . . . maybe not so much.

But as with your own family, which you did not choose to be born into, it is perfectly acceptable to parcel out your fucks to your in-laws according to what minimizes YOUR annoy (and maximizes your joy) while treating everyone in a respectful way.

When you inherit a bunch of new family members, there will be many line items added to your Fuck Budget. But if you think about it, these people inherited you too. And *your* religious values, and *your* political views, and *your* holiday traditions, and *your* aversion to dressing in matching turtlenecks for group photos.

When it comes to not giving a fuck, you might have more in common than you realize!

Which means that by practicing the NotSorry Method on your in-laws, you can ignite a chain reaction that culminates in an increase of happiness and harmony—and a decrease of fucks given—for all involved.

FAMILY STUFF I MAY OR MAY NOT
GIVE A FUCK ABOUT

(an inventory)

FAMILY STUFF I MAY OR MAY NOT GIVE A FUCK ABOUT

(an inventory)

FAMILY STUFF I MAY OR MAY NOT GIVE A FUCK ABOUT

(an inventory)

When dealing with family, sometimes you just want to throw up your hands and submit because: OBLIGATION and GUILT. I'm here to tell you, there are alternatives. Of course, I can't claim to absolve you of *all* guilty inclinations toward your family— that's what prescription benzodiazepines are for—but I can help you determine which aspects of family life are truly fuck-worthy and or nonnegotiable.

Remember: you are a *part* of your family, and you deserve to be happy too.

Consolidating your lists

By now, you've acquired the tools for deciding whether or not you give a fuck, and you've sorted all your potential fucks into manageable categories. You've waltzed around your mental barn and shone your metaphorical flashlight into its darkest corners, illuminating the fucks you've been collecting in there since . . . well, since before you picked up this journal.

Step 1 of the NotSorry Method—deciding what you don't give a fuck about—is well within your grasp.

You should have four exhaustive lists of stuff you may or may not give a fuck about from each of your four categories—the physical manifestation of your mental barn-decluttering tour.

Congrats, you've nearly made it to the fun part: crossing shit off!

First, a bit of light housekeeping. In the next few pages, I've provided space for you to copy out your lists into one master document for ease of reference. (It may seem onerous, but you can't skip this step, as it is a necessary precursor to the aforementioned fun part.)

MY MASTER LIST OF THINGS, WORK, FRIENDS, ACQUAINTANCES, STRANGERS, AND FAMILY-RELATED STUFF I MAY OR MAY NOT GIVE A FUCK ABOUT

(an inventory)

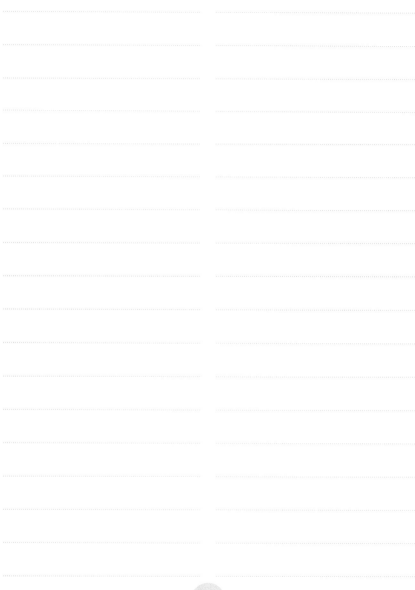

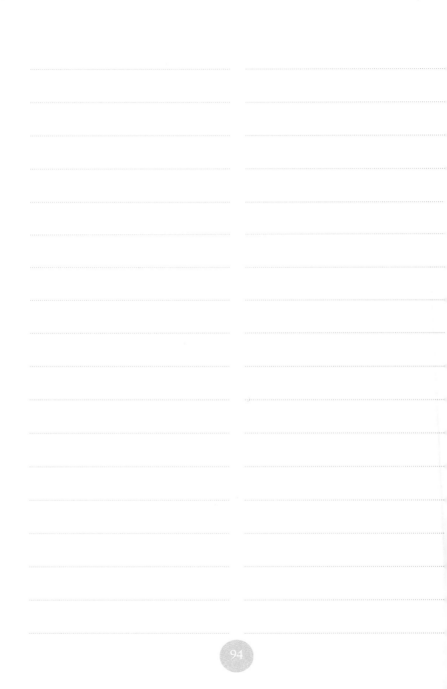

The fun part

———————

Now, grab that black marker I advised you to buy at the beginning of this process, and keep it handy as you review your master list, taking note of which fucks evoke those feelings of joy or annoy in your heart, your head, and your gut.

Remember as you go that "giving a fuck" is akin to spending your time, energy, and/or money on anything that made it onto one of your lists. **By crossing something out and NOT giving that fuck, you should GAIN more time, energy, and/or money to spend on everything else.** (Later, I'll give you an exercise that helps quantify those gains and will inspire you to hold your ground when you move forward into Step 2: not giving those fucks.) For now . . .

An agreeable fluttering in the chest or groin? Joy! Let your magic marker pass over these items like the Angel of Death passed over the firstborn sons of Israel.

Palpitations, dread, nausea? ANNOY ALERT. All of these are criteria for crossing off a fuck or three.

At this point in a physical decluttering spree, Marie Kondo would have you decide whether an object—a dress, a handbag, etc.—brings joy. If the answer is no, she instructs you to thank it for its service before discarding it. A little woo-woo, though I've got no problem with the general concept.

The thing is, I'm not so sure the items on your no-fucks list deserve thanks. I think they've drained your time, energy, and money for too long. So what I want you to do is this:

As your black marker hovers over those that annoy, touches down, and inscribes decisive strokes through the fucks you've finally decided to stop giving, you should utter a quiet, ceremonial "Fuck you" to each and every one.

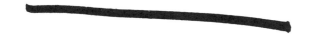

Feels good, doesn't it?

You're almost ready to take Step 2 and then start amassing magical, life-changing rewards! I'm delighted at how far you've come in such a short time. But hey, juuuuuust to make sure we're on the same page here, what about the things you didn't cross off your list?

Are you positive you don't want to rethink any of those?

Do not underestimate the drain of infrequent fuck-giving

There may be some annoying stuff that remains on your lists because you thought, *Eh, it's not like this comes up very often. Probably easier to just give the fuck and not deal with the fallout.*

Have I taught you nothing?!

If you continue to give your fucks willy-nilly to things that do not bring you joy, those fucks will continue to be expected of you. Like useless paperwork and *Keeping Up with the Kardashians* reruns, this is a vicious cycle.

Remember how a personal policy sets a precedent, in a positive way? Giving a fuck also sets a precedent—and makes it exponentially harder to stop giving that fuck in the future. If you've already committed to doing the time-consuming work of sorting your fucks into categories and making your lists and drawing up your Fuck Budgets, then why take the easy way out and continue to spend your fuck bucks on things that annoy, just because they only come around once or twice a year?

By that logic, you will spend every Christmas hungover and caroling in ten-degree weather wearing a stupid sweater.

Go back to your lists. Be honest with yourself and ruthless with your black marker. Trust me, it's worth it.

The power of honesty
cannot be overrated.
I can't tell you how
many *more* fucks you
wind up giving when
you try to beat around
the bush. God, even
that expression
sounds exhausting.

Giving a fuck

We've been dwelling on the negative for a while here to help get you to the heart of what you honestly don't give a fuck about. But the whole purpose of making these lists and crossing out things that threaten to overdraw your Fuck Budget is to reveal the ones that *are* worthy. And to create more time and emotional space to preserve and pursue those relationships and activities and give them the fucks they deserve.

That's the life-changing magic in a nutshell.

If you consulted the flowchart, worked your steps, and determined that there are indeed things on your lists that you give a fuck about, then go ahead, give them! Giving a fuck is easy. You don't need me for that. (Though I thank you for your patronage.)

For everything else, it's time to put Step 2 of the NotSorry Method—not giving a fuck—into action.

STEP 2:

DON'T GIVE A
FUCK ABOUT
THOSE THINGS.

FUQs
(Frequently Uttered Questions)

Oh, like you've never made a bad pun before. Go ahead, judge me. Guess what I don't give???

I thought it would be helpful at this juncture to address some of the most common questions I receive when I talk to people about the NotSorry Method—questions that I'm pretty sure are popping into your head even as you gleefully cross items off of your various lists. You've made some big decisions, but actually not giving a fuck? That's easier fantasized about in the comfort of your own mind than said out loud at Shabbat dinner.

I know how it is—believe me—but my advice is to harness the fever while it's burning hot within you. No time like the present to get your fucks in order and start living your best life!

On that note, here are some FUQs to help you feel better about taking Step 2.

Q: Telling people I don't give a fuck feels inherently impolite. Don't you think it's kind of rude?

A: Well, if the F-word gives you pause, you don't actually have to say it out loud. You can communicate your decision to not spend your time, energy, or money on something in a totally G-rated fashion (e.g., "I confess I don't share your opinion on X, but you do you!"). I don't think it's as much fun, but that's for me to give a fuck about, not you.

Q: I'm worried that if I stop giving a fuck about too many things, I'm going to like it so much that I become a lazy sack of shit with nothing and nobody to live for.

A: It's a legitimate concern, but the goal of the NotSorry Method is *not* actually to get to #ZeroFucks (an amusing if impractical hash tag). It's to pare away the fucks that don't bring you joy, *paving* the way for the fucks that do.

Q: If not giving a fuck is supposed to be so liberating, why does it feel so uncomfortable?

A: Not wearing clothes is liberating too. But it can also be uncomfortable because society isn't ready for this jelly. All it takes is a little confidence (and a little baby powder); you'll see.

Q: Even though everything you've said makes perfect sense [Why, thank you!], I just know I'm not going to get away with giving fewer fucks when it comes to ....

A: All I can say is, you won't know until you try. And it's worked out pretty well for me, so . . .

Q: What if I decide I don't give a fuck about something, and then I don't give the fuck, and then I regret it?

A: Now you're just stalling.

Q: I wouldn't want people to tell me they didn't give a fuck about something that was important to *me*, so how can I tell them I don't give a fuck about something that's important to *them*?

A: Let me throw it back at you in a different way. Would you want people to feel obligated and/or guilted into doing something for you that you *knew* they didn't want to do? The answer to THAT question should always be no, or you're the asshole. And you wouldn't know that they felt this way unless they were comfortable telling you, and vice versa. This is precisely how taking Step 2 unlocks life-changing magic for EVERYONE.

Look at you, on the cusp of not giving a fuck! The view from up here is pretty special, isn't it?

In the first half of the journal, you learned to qualify the fucks you give based on whether they annoy or bring joy. You learned to quantify them based on whether they fit into your Fuck Budget. And you've been introduced to the tools and perspective—namely, feelings, opinions, honesty, and politeness—with which to make those calculations.

You made all those lists and you decided which fucks you just don't want to give. Maybe you even had to buy a new black marker because your first one ran out of ink. (I've seen it happen.) I congratulate you.

But it's about to get so much better, because now you're actually going to STOP GIVING A FUCK.

Excited? Yay!

Nervous? Don't worry; I was too. I got over it.

And the next exercise is sure to help YOU get over it too.

A fuck not given is something gained

As you know, time, energy, and money are the resources you regain by ceasing to give a fuck. And it's quite useful to keep them foremost in your mind when gearing up to actually not give those fucks—aka when preparing yourself to say no to the people, things, events, tasks, and obligations that no longer deserve a place of honor in your Fuck Budget.

Visualizing your gains releases endorphins into your brain. And in my professional opinion, endorphins are magic. With this in mind, give those knuckles a nice cracking and sharpen up your pencil, because it's time to make another list.

Hey, I said "lists *galore*" and I meant it.

In the next few pages, we're going to resurrect a few of those not-given fucks from beneath their black marker shroud.

NOTE: This is not an effort to make you second-guess your discarding decisions. On the contrary, we're doing it to help you visualize all of the gains you stand to make when you proceed with Step 2.

Not giving a fuck requires preparation and finesse. You need to articulate your fucks to *yourself*—by touring your mental barn and making your lists and balancing your Fuck Budget—then, act accordingly.

WHAT'S IN IT FOR ME?: AN EXERCISE

Go back to your master list from page 89 and pull **5–10* THINGS** about which you've decided you do not give a fuck. (I realize it might be hard to see them through the heavy tread of your marker, but I have a feeling they're pretty fresh in your mind.)

Consider each item carefully, and ask yourself, *When I stop giving my fucks to this, what will I gain?*

Mark a little *T* next to all the fucks not given that will result in more time for you to spend as you wish. Then do an *E* for energy, and, finally, an *M* for money.

5–10 FUCKS I NO LONGER GIVE
(THINGS)

Now we're going to plug each fuck you've decided not to give into the Venn diagram on the next page.

---

* If, by now, you do not have a minimum of five things in your mental barn about which you no longer give a fuck, you either did not need this journal, or you're not doing it right.

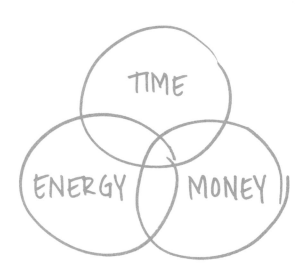

Some items will fall in just one segment of the diagram, some in various sections of $T + E$ or $E + M$, etc. And, obviously, it's not giving those fucks situated smack in the middle of where $T + E + M$ intersect that will free you up in the most delightful ways possible.

To see what the finished exercise should look like, turn the page for an example of ten things that I, personally, do not give a fuck about, and where they fall in my diagram.

10 THINGS ABOUT WHICH I, PERSONALLY, DO NOT GIVE A FUCK

What Other People Think. Remember: This one is nonnegotiable. All fucks stem from here.

Having a "bikini body." Oh good God, the day I stopped giving a fuck about how I looked in a bathing suit, it was like a litter of kittens in black leotards had tumbled down from heaven to perform "All the Single Ladies" for the sole enjoyment of my thighs and belly. Magical!

Basketball. I have never enjoyed or understood basketball.

Being a morning person. For most of my life I was ashamed of being useless in the early hours and not wanting to schedule anything before noon. Society really seems to value morning people and look down on those of us who don't (or can't) fall in line. Once I embraced the freelance life, I stopped giving a fuck about being a morning person once and for all. Snack on it, morning people.

Taylor Swift.* Everybody be all, "Tay-Tay!" and I'm like, "Nope."

---

* Technically she is a human whom I do not know personally, so she could go in the "STRANGERS" category, but I think of her as more of a concept. My barn, my rules.

Iceland. I'm sure Iceland is a beautiful country, but every time someone starts telling me about plans for their once-in-a-lifetime trip to Iceland, or about how much fun they had in Iceland, or that "the majority of Icelanders believe in elves!" my eyes start glazing over like I'm at a Knicks game.

Calculus. This may have been my earliest recorded instance of not giving a fuck. My high-school guidance counselor insisted that I had to take this class in order to have any hope of getting into a good college. I did not take the class, and I *did* get into Harvard. You can't argue with those results.

Feigning sincerity. I am the embodiment of "If you don't have anything nice to say, don't say anything at all." I just don't give a fuck about faking it.

Passwords. I used to have so much anxiety about personal security, but then I read a number of articles by experts that suggest we're all one pimply Slavic teenager away from getting hacked anyway, so I decided I should probably stop giving a fuck about devising a different Alan Turing-approved crypto phrase for my Gap, Ann Taylor, and Victoria's Secret accounts. So far, so good.

Google Plus. As of this writing, even Google doesn't give a fuck about Google Plus anymore. Never tried it, myself. #NotSorry.

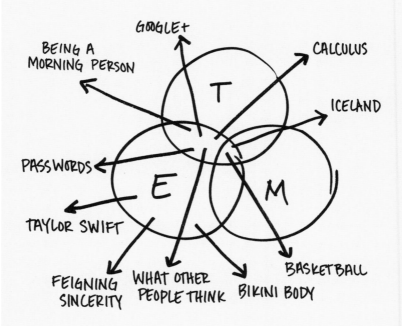

GOOGLE+

BEING A
MORNING PERSON

CALCULUS

ICELAND

T

PASSWORDS

E

M

TAYLOR SWIFT

FEIGNING
SINCERITY

WHAT OTHER
PEOPLE THINK

BIKINI BODY

BASKETBALL

As you can see, my diagram is heavy on time and energy gains, less heavy on monetary ones. This makes sense because I value my time highly—it is, after all, the very definition of a finite resource, and I am perhaps more preoccupied with my own mortality than the average bear. In my view, additional money can at least *potentially* be earned or borrowed if need be; whereas there is no such thing as "borrowed time." (Although I'm sure if American Express could figure that one out at 16.9% interest, they would.)

But, hey, different strokes for different folks! It doesn't really matter *which* resources are more valuable to you when doing this exercise, just that you learn to recognize them— and get that much more fired up about taking them back.

If you haven't already done so, go back to page 109 and fill in your diagram. Then move through the other Categories of Potential Fuck-giving, visualizing your gains as you go.

5–10 FUCKS I NO LONGER GIVE
(WORK)

....

....

....

....

....

BY NOT GIVING THESE FUCKS, I WILL GAIN:

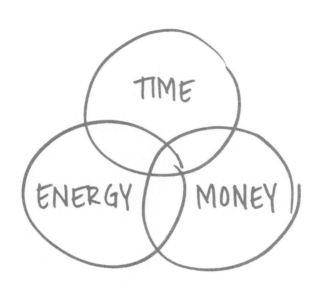

5–10 FUCKS I NO LONGER GIVE
(FRIENDS, ACQUAINTANCES,
AND STRANGERS)

BY NOT GIVING THESE FUCKS,
I WILL GAIN:

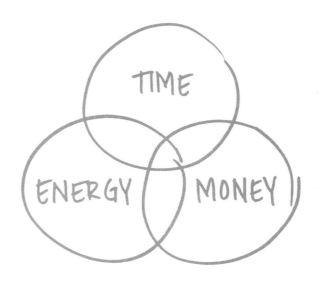

5–10 FUCKS I NO LONGER GIVE
(FAMILY)

BY NOT GIVING THESE FUCKS, I WILL GAIN:

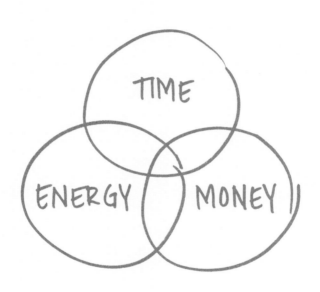

Planning and execution

Whew! Now that you've decluttered your mental barn and psyched yourself up by visualizing all the time, energy, and money you're going to gain by giving fewer, better fucks, you are officially IN IT TO WIN IT (life, that is).

Seriously, I can smell your endorphins from here.

To keep up your momentum without overtaxing your newly liberated fuck muscles, I'm going to lay out a program designed to get you giving fewer, better fucks as easily and seamlessly as possible.

The next section of the journal is divided into three levels of EASY, MEDIUM-TOUGH, and HARD fucks to stop giving. I'll give you examples of each, and then you'll have space to write down your own—taken straight from your lists—along with your plans for not giving them, and ultimately, the *results* of not having given them.

This way, if things don't work out as you hoped, you can revisit your strategy (and your flowchart), find the weak links in your planning and/or execution, and try again.

Practice makes perfect, motherfuckers.

Threat level yellow: easy fucks to stop giving

We'll start with the stuff that affects only you, thereby taking Step 2 of the NotSorry Method without even having to worry about hurting other people's feelings (which, as you may know, can be *supremely* inconvenient). You might not even need to be polite. In fact, all you really have to be is honest—with yourself. For example:

Don't give a fuck about your Facebook friend's constant drama? "Unfollow" is one of the easiest ways to not give a fuck ever invented. None of the confrontation of "Unfriend" and all of the benefits.

Don't give a fuck about wrinkles? Stop spending money on lotions and serums, time applying them to your face, and energy worrying about the visible signs of aging, which—spoiler alert—are actually impossible to counteract unless your name is Christie Brinkley. Hot damn, she looks good.

Don't give a fuck about understanding the stock market? Stop banging your head against the *Wall Street Journal* just to make yourself sound knowledgeable at dinner parties. Instead, use that time to become an expert on something that is truly meaningful to you—perhaps small-batch bourbon?—and let someone else field all the stock tips for your friend group.

How I'm going to do it:

Results:

How I'm going to do it:

Results:

How I'm going to do it:

Results:

How I'm going to do it:

Results:

How I'm going to do it:

Results:

How I'm going to do it:

Results:

How I'm going to do it:

Results:

How I'm going to do it:

Results:

How I'm going to do it:

Results:

How I'm going to do it:

Results:

How I'm going to do it:

Results:

_____

How I'm going to do it:

Results:

How I'm going to do it:

Results:

_____

How I'm going to do it:

Results:

How I'm going to do it:

Results:

I've mentioned repeatedly that honesty and politeness are the keys to not giving a fuck without being an asshole. You should always be keeping these principles in mind.

HOWEVER, I acknowledge that when the going gets tough, you may need to get a little, shall we say, flexible.

Honesty is *usually* the best policy. It allows you to say things like "I'm sorry, I don't have time to read your self-published novel about gnomes, but I wish you all the best with it" or "I don't like tea." Simple and direct and, if delivered politely, very effective.

Not hurting people's feeling *and* not getting caught in a lie is the purest form of NotSorry. You have nothing to agonize over OR apologize for.

But we all know there are times when you've charted your most polite and honest course of action, yet implementing Step 2 feels . . . icky. The good news is, if you're feeling that "ick" factor, it means you're not an asshole. They never get the jitters.

If you have a hunch that full-blown honesty is NOT, in fact, the best policy, you can fudge it a little. I won't tell.

TIMES WHEN FULL-BLOWN HONESTY IS PERHAPS NOT THE BEST POLICY

When it involves someone else's cooking

When you don't want to have to talk to
anyone's therapist about it

When Santa and small children are part of the equation

When dealing with a pregnant woman

When dealing with your mother-in-law

When dealing with your pregnant mother-in-law

Okay, now let's move on to stuff that represents an unreasonable drain on your Fuck Budget and that you have every right to discard—but that also may affect other people and require a conversation about opinions and/or feelings. Such as:

Don't give a fuck that your forty-year-old friend has to move apartments tomorrow and is asking for helpers "in exchange for beer"? Pure honesty ("I can't be responsible for your failings as an adult") may not be the best policy here, but you can still politely beg off, citing some vague work commitment. After all, what does he know about work commitments?

Don't give a fuck about promoting synergy in the workplace? At first you might worry that your boss is going to call you out on this one, but rest assured, synergy is exceedingly difficult to quantify and your lack of fucks won't change that. Reserve this creative energy for something that will benefit YOU— like devising the winning bracket in the office sweepstake.

Don't give a fuck about your coworker's decision to procreate? It's as easy as not putting any money in that Diapers.com gift-card envelope they're passing around the office. Worried that people will think you're cheap? Then you need to stop giving a fuck about what other people think.

How I'm going to do it:

Results:

How I'm going to do it:

Results:

How I'm going to do it:

Results:

How I'm going to do it:

Results:

YOU
DO
YOU

I just want to pause for a second to make sure you know that *The Life-Changing Magic of Not Giving a Fuck Journal* is meant to be aspirational and inspirational—not tyrannical—in its teachings. You're allowed to change your mind, revise your personal policies, and reallocate accordingly.

You've heard of a crime of opportunity? Well, you might commit a fuck of opportunity.

Like, I really, truly don't give a fuck about karaoke, but if I'm already at the bar and someone dangles that microphone in my face and I'm lubed up with enough Bacardi to anesthetize a pony, well . . . things happen. As you well know if you've ever witnessed me perform "Faith" or "Like a Virgin" under the twin influences of rum punch and peer pressure.

Anyway, all I'm saying is that in the heat of the moment, you might find yourself giving an unexpected fuck and it might even bring you joy. Fun!

Or at least bring the people watching you make a fool of yourself some joy, which isn't the worst thing you can do for your fellow man every once in a while.

How I'm going to do it:

Results:

How I'm going to do it:

Results:

How I'm going to do it:

Results:

How I'm going to do it:

Results:

How I'm going to do it:

Results:

How I'm going to do it:

Results:

How I'm going to do it:

Results:

_____

How I'm going to do it:

Results:

How I'm going to do it:

Results:

How I'm going to do it:

Results:

How I'm going to do it:

Results:

A pep talk

Even after you've made your decisions about which fucks not to give, and you've diagrammed your lists and succeeded with the easy-to-medium-tough stuff, you may be tempted to backslide a little. It's common. No worries! Like the birth control pill, the NotSorry Method is revolutionary but not 100 percent foolproof. If you find yourself experiencing morning-after nausea, keep in mind: it's all part of the process.

For example, let's say your coworker, Tim, is having a karaoke birthday party. A quick glance through your lists reveals that you don't give a fuck about karaoke, or Tim, or maybe birthday parties in general. In fact, you're quite sure that no one in your office wants to go to this party, but now that you've been using your trusty journal, you're the only one brave enough to say so. You implement Step 2, RSVP no, and skip the party.

Success!

But the next day, you're not so sure you did the right thing . . .

. . . Maybe Tim or others are giving you the cold shoulder. (Focus: Do you give a fuck about what they think?) You start to get uncomfortable. You begin to question your decision to not have given a fuck about your coworker and his party. You spend a few more fuck bucks just worrying about it.

Stop right there.

It is important not to confuse this feeling with those of regret or shame. You made the right decision. For God's sake, they sang an *entire* Kenny Chesney album! That's not a twinge of regret you are experiencing; that's FREEDOM with a side of pity for the rest of your coworkers—about most of whose opinions you will, eventually, stop giving a fuck.

Carry on.

Threat level red:
the hardest fucks to stop giving

These fucks will require all your tools plus a fair amount of self-possession and maybe a personal policy or two. They involve other people, have high potential for hurting feelings/being an asshole, and are often socially unacceptable. In other words, what the NotSorry Method was invented for.

Don't give a fuck about extended-family weddings, graduations, and similar events? These things are usually planned fairly far in advance. That's how they get you. I recommend another visualization exercise: Before you blithely check the "Yes" box on the RSVP card, making a dent in your Fuck Budget before the reality of the consequences can sink in, think about how you're likely to feel *on that day*—or, worse, the night before, when you're in line at airport security on your way to third cousin Barry's *Star Wars*-themed wedding in Pittsburgh. As Yoda might say, "In a dark place we find ourselves, and a little more knowledge lights our way." If you can access that deep reservoir of despair *before* you RSVP, you're going to save yourself days (weeks? months?) of regret and anxiety leading up to the event and thousands of dollars in airfare and hotels. Simply check "RSVP Regrets" on the response card and send a gift. Perhaps a nice Death Star cutting board?

Don't give a fuck about your friends' children? First, you need to make it clear that it's not just *their* children—it's all children! In that way, it's somewhat of a personal policy. (And if you're a parent yourself, "all children except mine" works too.) However, literally saying the words "I do not give a fuck about your children" is unlikely to yield positive results. You may never have to deal with those kids again, but you've also probably lost a friend. Assuming you want to keep your friends and not hurt their feelings—but NOT be expected to attend functions where the guest of honor is a toddler or ever, *under any circumstances*, be asked to babysit—then you have to add a heaping helping of politeness in with that honesty. An occasional lollipop or *So cute!* shout-out on social media can be very effective. It's the whole "spoonful of sugar helps the medicine go down" philosophy. (Mary Poppins: NotSorry since 1934.)

Don't give a fuck about puppies? Yeah, good luck with that.

How I'm going to do it:

Results:

How I'm going to do it:

Results:

How I'm going to do it:

Results:

How I'm going to do it:

Results:

How I'm going to do it:

Results:

How I'm going to do it:

Results:

Getting cold feet?
Revisit your personal policies!

How I'm going to do it:

Results:

How I'm going to do it:

Results:

How I'm going to do it:

Results:

How I'm going to do it:

Results:

How I'm going to do it:

Results:

How I'm going to do it:

Results:

How I'm going to do it:

Results:

How I'm going to do it:

Results:

How I'm going to do it:

Results:

Fuck the haters

In the vein of that very first admonition I handed
down re: not giving a fuck about what other people
think, I wanted to pay special attention to a subset of
those people, aka the haters. At this point in your study
of the NotSorry Method, you're likely to encounter a
few of them, and you need to be prepared. These people
are, at the least, baffled, and at the most, grievously
offended by your life decisions. For whatever reason,
they just don't have the desire or wherewithal to accept
NotSorry into their lives. And that's okay! But you
don't have to be weighed down by their narrow-
mindedness or insecurity. Your life is great
and getting better every day.
Fuck the haters!

Performance bonuses

Are there some fucks you're having trouble just not giving? Family-related, perhaps? I get it, which is why I have another trick for making the best out of a less-than-ideal situation: built-in performance bonuses!

For example, if you just can't avoid a family holiday get-together, you *can* schedule a massage for the day after so you have something to look forward to. Even better, request the massage as your holiday gift so your family is essentially paying you back for the fuck you gave. Sneaky.

(#ProTip: Upgrading to first class on the flight home is also an effective, if wildly expensive, balm for the enervating family gathering.)

Or if you have to sit through your mother's Rotary luncheon at which she's being honored for outstanding service to the community that you grew up in and fled immediately upon turning eighteen, liberate one of the honoree's Percocets from the medicine cabinet beforehand. You're about to earn it.

And if you can't realistically opt out of the group photo, resolve to wear your kinkiest or most hilarious undergarments that day and I guarantee you the whole process will be more bearable. Plus, when the pic starts clogging your Facebook feed with comments like *Beautiful family!!!!* and *OMG they're so grown up!* you will take secret pleasure in knowing you were wearing your POISON PARTIED HERE thong.*

Use the next couple of pages to make a list of potential bonuses with which you could motivate/reward yourself in times of need.

Aim high! You're gonna need 'em.

* I may or may not be the proud owner of a POISON PARTIED HERE thong.

PERFORMANCE BONUSES

PERFORMANCE BONUSES

SHOW ME WHAT YOU GOT: THE FINAL EXERCISE

Earlier, we visualized your *potential* gains to get you psyched up for taking Step 2. Now that you have (presumably) stopped giving quite a few fucks, let's record your *actual* gains.

This is gonna be good.

TIME

The first thing people tend to get back when they put their fucks in order is TIME. Time to meditate quietly on the toilet instead of rushing to get on a conference call; time to cultivate that prizewinning fudge recipe on a Sunday afternoon instead of reading *Moby-Dick* for your book club (who picked that?); time to spend with a loved one instead of, well, time to spend with some random fuckers you don't even like.

What have you gained thus far in terms of time? Three hours? Ten minutes? One weekend a month? I smell a list coming on!

TIME I HAVE GAINED BY
NOT GIVING A FUCK

Activity   Benefit

Example:

Not watching the VMAs   2 hours

ENERGY

The second thing the NotSorry Method returns to you is ENERGY. That can be as simple as taking a blessed nap or as complex as conserving energy by not doing one activity—that CrossFit class you only signed up for because your friend pressured you into it—and then *expending* it on something you'd rather be doing, like finally cleaning out your car because it's starting to smell like you imagine that lady from *The Goonies* does. Not giving a fuck dramatically increases your energy reserves day in and day out.

What have you been using all your newfound energy on?

ENERGY I HAVE GAINED BY
NOT GIVING A FUCK

Activity	Benefit
Example:	
Not getting wasted at margarita Mondays with coworkers	The will to live on Tuesday

MONEY

Last but not least is MONEY. As the American humorist and performer Will Rogers once said, "Too many people spend money they haven't earned to buy things they don't want to impress people that they don't like." Sing it, sister!

And because money is so easily quantified, it is especially satisfying when you apply the NotSorry Method and it results in tangible financial gains. If you stopped giving a fuck about, say, designer clothes—in part because you've stopped giving a fuck about what other people think—you could stand to save hundreds or thousands of dollars in any given year. I know so many women who feel pressured to fit in by way of overspending on name-brand labels when clothes at half or even less the price would look good and make them perfectly happy.

Or maybe you're a suburbanite who stopped giving a fuck about traveling every Sunday to your six-year-old nephew's soccer games—let's just say he's unlikely to go pro and snag you free tickets to the 2034 World Cup. Not only are you saving time and energy, you're saving gas money. That $2.50 a gallon really adds up, and Auntie needs a new pair of off-brand sunglasses.

Total it up!

MONEY I HAVE GAINED BY
NOT GIVING A FUCK

Activity	Benefit
Example:	
Not going to that Vegas bachelor party	$1,000*

---

* Occasionally you have to spend *some* money to be a good friend and gain peace of mind. In this case you might want to send a stripper or maybe a singing telegram, so the formula is $ SAVED ($1,000)-COMPENSATORY $ SPENT ($200 on stripper/ singing telegram) = NET SAVINGS ($800). Still not bad!

The path to living your
best life is paved with
reclaimed hours,
newfound verve,
and cold hard cash.

Congratufuckinglations, you did it!

If you made it this far, you must have really wanted to make a change. You were fed up with looking at your life as a series of obligations to be met, people to tolerate, and calendar squares to be desperately reshuffled until a blessed wild card in the form of a free afternoon rose to the top.

Or maybe this journal was a gift from a friend, in which case they were probably trying to tell you something, and good on you for listening.

Whatever the path that brought you here, by now you know that your best life is well within your grasp—and the parameters of your Fuck Budget. I hope you'll find *The Life-Changing Magic of Not Giving a Fuck Journal* a useful tool to return to in times of need, whenever things, work, friends, acquaintances, strangers, and family begin to encroach on the newly-tidied confines of your mental barn.

Just remember: be honest, be polite, don't be an asshole, and you'll be fine.

STOP GIVING A FUCK

AND START LIVING YOUR BEST LIFE!

First published in Great Britain in 2020 by

Quercus Editions Ltd
Carmelite House
50 Victoria Embankment
London EC4Y 0DZ

An Hachette UK company

A CIP catalogue record for this book is available from the British Library.

ISBN 978 1 52940 633 7

Some material previously published in *The Life-Changing Magic of Not Giving a F**k*, also by Sarah Knight.

Illustrations and hand lettering by Lauren Harms

This book is not approved, endorsed or authorized by Marie Kondo or her publishers.

10 9 8 7 6 5 4 3

Designed and typeset by Rich Carr

Printed and bound in China by C&C Offset Printing Co., Ltd.

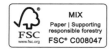

MIX
Paper | Supporting
responsible forestry
FSC® C008047